The Book of Buddhas

Other books by Binkey Kok Publications bv

Eva Rudy Jansen
Singing Bowls
A Practical Handbook of Instruction and Use
ISBN 90-74597-01-7

Ab Williams
The Complete Book of Chinese Health Balls
Background and Use of the Health Balls
ISBN 90-74597-28-9

Eva Rudy Jansen
The Book of Hindu Imagery
The Gods and their Symbols
ISBN 90-74597-07-6 PBK
ISBN 90-74597-10-6 CLOTH

Dirk Schellberg
Didgeridoo
Ritual Origins and Playing Techniques
ISBN 90-74597-13-0

George Hulskramer
The Life of Buddha
From Prince Siddhartha to Buddha
ISBN 90-74597-17-3

Töm Klöwer
The Joy of Drumming
Drums and Percussion Instruments from around the World
ISBN 90-74597-13-9

Eva Rudy Jansen

The Book of Buddhas

**Ritual symbolism used
on Buddhist Statuary and Ritual Objects**

Binkey Kok Publications bv, Havelte, Holland

CIP-DATA KONINKLIJKE BIBLIOTHEEK, DEN HAAG

Jansen, Eva Rudy

The book of Buddhas : ritual symbolism used on Buddhist
statuary and ritual objects / Eva Rudy Jansen ; [ill.
Bert Wieringa ; transl. from the Dutch by Tony Langam...
et al.]. − Diever : Binkey Kok. − Ill.
Transl. of: Het Boeddha-boekje : Boeddha's, godheden en
rituele symbolen. − Diever : Binkey Kok, 1990. − With
index.
ISBN 90-74597-02-5
Subject heading: Buddhism.

Published and © by Binkey Kok Publications bv
Havelte, Holland
www.binkeykok.com
e-mail: info@binkeykok.com

Printed and bound in the Netherlands.
Lay-out: Eva Rudy Jansen
Cover design: Jaap Koning.

Distributed in the U.S.A. by Samuel Weiser Inc., Box 612, York Beach,
Maine 03910-0612
Orderphone: 1-800-423-7087

© 1990 by Binkey Kok.
© Second printing 1994 by Binkey Kok.
© Third printing 1995 by Binkey Kok.
© Fourth printing 1997 by Binkey Kok.
© Fifth printing 1998 by Binkey Kok Publications bv
© Sixth printing 1999 by Binkey Kok Publications bv
© Seventh printing 2000 by Binkey Kok Publications bv
© Eight printing 2001 by Binkey Kok Publications bv
© Nineth printing 2004 by Binkey Kok Publications bv

To

Samantabhadra
the Complete God

Manjusri
the Lord of Inspiration

and

Ganesh
the impartial Protector of all Wisdom

Contents

Foreword

In the course of time, many different views have evolved on Buddhism, and countless works have been written. A true insight can only be obtained after many years of study and meditation; or after many lives ...

Therefore it is absolutely impossible to give a complete, or even completely accurate survey of Buddhist philosophy in such a small booklet as this. In addition, the approach adopted in this book of providing a survey of the images representing a number of visual elements in certain schools of Buddhism, means that the text is also geared to this visual aspect.

Even for the everyday followers of these schools of Buddhism themselves, the wealth of external forms readily lends itself to viewing the figures, each with their own name and function, only as gods and holy men with their 'own' life, who can be called upon to offer their services to mortal 'unredeemed' man.

At one level, it certainly works in this way, but at another level, all these images are actually mirrors, aspects and faculties inherent in everyone, which have been made manifest. By giving them their own existence and form, it is easier to recognize and understand these aspects. However, the ultimate goal is always to turn the insight obtained in this way inwards, where it leads to self-knowledge and self-awareness, and thus to a release from the constricting bonds of the conditioning of the mind which trap every thinking being. It is only when you break through this conditioning that there is room for liberating enlightenment. Viewed in this way,

Buddhism can be seen as a system that is based on profound psychological insight.

As far as possible, this booklet tries to ensure that an aspect of this 'internal' side remains visible. In this respect the author is particularly grateful to Erik Bruijn, whose book, 'Tantra, Yoga and Meditation' (published by Ankh-Hermes b.v., Deventer 1980), gave support on this inner path.

Structure of the book

Tibetan Buddhists follow a strict ritual order in which they invoke or depict beings. This order is as follows (for invocation, from the first to the last, and for depicting, in the reverse order):

1. Gurus
2. Yidams
3. Buddhas
4. Bodhisattvas
5. Dakas, dakinis, yoginis
6. Dharmapalas
7. Yakshas
8. Gods and goddesses of prosperity and wealth
9. Other deities

I have not used the above order in this book for the description of these beings. It seemed more appropriate for the uninitiated to begin with the Buddha figures, and then progress to the other beings and manifestations. In doing this, the most logical order possible was adopted, but it remains the logic of the author.

Introduction

About 2,500 years ago Gautama Siddhartha, a man who had renounced his princely title to lead a life of meditation, was sitting under a tree and realized what was the cause of suffering in the world. From that moment he was Buddha, and his teachings have become a 'world religion', although Buddhism is not essentially concerned with the question of the existence of an omnipotent god. In Buddhism, man and everything that takes place in man is central. The insight into suffering which Gautama achieved in his condition of supreme enlightenment under the 'bodhi tree' ('bodhi' means enlightenment) is called the Four Noble Truths. These truths are:

1. Suffering, as a synonym for the bonds of earthly existence and not being freed from the chain of rebirth;
2. The origin of suffering, i.e., the desire for joy, lust and possession;
3. The elimination of suffering, i.e., the destruction of desire, hatred and ignorance;
4. The road to the elimination of suffering in the form of the "Noble Eightfold Path". This path entails:
   1. the right understanding,
   2. the right attitude of mind,
   3. the right speech,
   4. the right action,
   5. the right conduct,
   6. the right effort,
   7. the right attention,
   8. the right meditation.

Everyone can release himself from the inner bonds of matter and suffering, and thus from suffering itself, and be enlightened, by following this Path and by seeking refuge with 'The Three Jewels', viz., Buddha – as an historical figure and principle of enlightenment; Dharma – the teaching and also the cosmic law; and Sangha – the community both of the monks and of those who have achieved the cosmic law.

Three times the historical Buddha turned the 'Wheel of Law', i.e., made a speech in which he explained his teachings, successively appealing to three different levels of understanding. This resulted in three different disciplines known as 'The Three Vehicles':

1. *Hinayana* – the 'Small Vehicle', also known as Theradava. This 'basic doctrine' assumes that every person can attain enlightenment for himself alone by means of self-discipline, through many lives. To do this, he must aim to follow the Four Truths and the Eightfold Path. His goal is to reach Nirvana, the place where all suffering is resolved.

2. *Mahayana* – the 'Large Vehicle', also known as Bodhistvayana. This 'middle doctrine' assumes that enlightenment can only be attained with help from outside. Training and teaching by an enlightened teacher, as well as faith and devotion, and the help of the timeless, transcendental Bodhisattvas, lead to buddhahood. It is a selfless path because it is aimed at enlightenment for all living creatures together and total enlightenment is deferred until that moment has come. The goal is Tatatha, non-dualism, the absolute void.

3. *Vajrayana* – the 'Diamond Vehicle', also known as Tantrayana. This 'final doctrine' is based on the idea that every being is a potential Buddha. However, he is not aware of this because of the thick mist of ignorance and confusion which obscures his spirit. This is the cause of suffering. It is possible to dispel this mist with insight and right action, and attain a state of great salvation (Mahasubbha). For this purpose the spirit must be trained and aimed at that single goal. The specific Tantric path is based on the idea that enlightenment can be attained in a single lifetime, and views every element in existence as a means to this goal. The body and the mind, passions and desires, are no more than forms of energy which can be used by directing them towards the goal of enlightenment.

Both the language and iconography of Mahayana and Vajrayana are rich in imagery and symbolism. Every aspect of enlightenment is represented in one of the transcendental Buddhas and Bodhisattvas, and in the divine figures often taken over from older religions. In countries such as Nepal and Tibet, magnificent works of art are produced especially for this purpose. Contemplating these figures is an exercise in meditation to establish inner contact with the aspect that is represented. Each gesture, each position and each individual attribute has a symbolic significance.

Part 1

The Three Mysteries

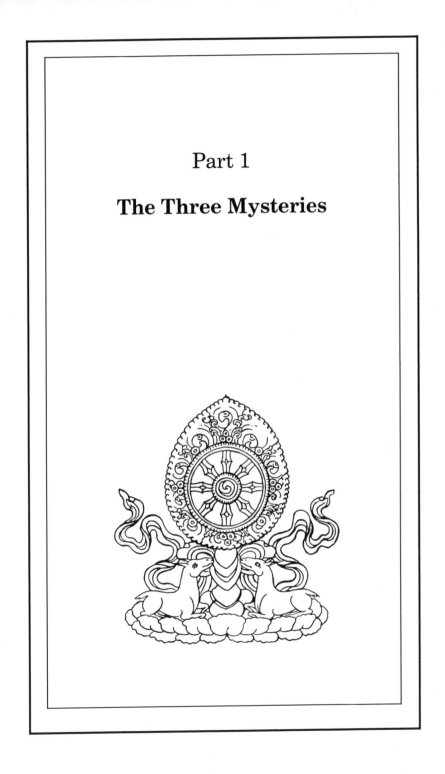

The Three Mysteries

In Tantric meditationexercises the forces of the spirit, speech, and the body ('Triguya', or the Three Mysteries), are directed at the one and only goal: enlightenment. The expedients to attain this purpose are mandalas (spirit), mantras (speech), and mudras and asanas (body).

Mandala
A ritual diagram which shows the structure as well as the unity of both the microcosm and macrocosm of the inner and outer world. Thus it is a practical aid on the path to enlightenment. The basic shape is that of a temple or palace, with doors at the four points of the compass. The transcendental inhabitant of the mandala dwells at the centre. All the components, such as symbols, attributes, deities, and lesser gods are shown on the mandala in accordance with a strict ritual; the making of the mandala is the meditation exercise.

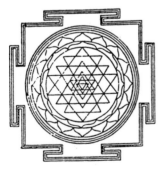

Yantra
An abstract mandala shape, a diagram of inter-connected lines used in meditation for concentrating the visualized energy. There are different sorts of yantras which can be made from different materials, e.g., rock crystal. Depicted here is the Sri yantra, or 'Great Yantra'.

Mantra
A sound or word symbol that is spoken aloud or silently in meditation. The mantra helps to achieve a connection with the deeper layers of consciousness. The mantra shown here is the Tibetan mantra 'OM MANI PADME HUM', the devotional formula for 'the Jewel in the Lotus', Avalokitesvara.

ཨོཾ་མ་ཎི་པ་དྨེ་ཧཱུྃ

Mudra
A symbolic position of the hand. The mudra is a physical expression of a particular energy. Mudras are used in illustrations, but also as an aid in meditation to release the relevant energies in the person practising these gestures.

Asana
A ritual position of the body with the same purpose as the mudra. The word asana is also used to indicate the pedestal on which the represented figure is seated or standing.

Mudras

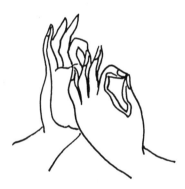

Dharmachakra
The gesture of Teaching, usually interpreted as: turning the Wheel of Law. The hands are held level with the heart, the thumbs and index fingers form circles.

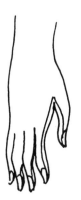

Bhumisparsa
Touching the earth as Gautama did, to invoke the earth as a witness to the truth of his words.

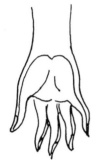

Varada
Fulfillment of all wishes; the gesture of Charity.

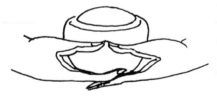

Dhyana
The gesture of absolute balance, of meditation. The hands are relaxed in the lap, and the tips of the thumbs and fingers touch each other. When depicted with a begging bowl, this is a sign of the Head of an Order.

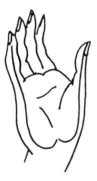

Abhaya
Gesture of reassurance, blessing and protection. 'Do not fear'.

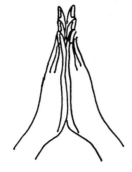

Namaskara
Gesture of greeting, prayer and adoration. Buddhas no longer make this gesture because they do not have to show devotion for anything.

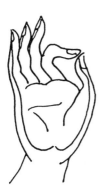

Vitarka
Intellectual argument, discussion. The circle formed by the thumb and index finger is the sign of the 'Wheel of Law'.

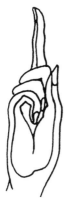

Tarjani
Threat, warning. The extended index finger is pointed at the opponent.

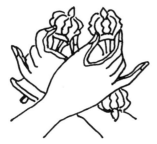

Vajrahumkara
This gesture, with ghanta and vajra (see p. 15-16), shows the symbolic significance of these two attributes: path and purpose are one.

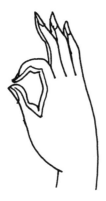

Jnana
Teaching. The hand is held at chest level and the thumb and index finger again form the 'Wheel of Law'.

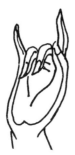

Karana
Gesture with which demons are expelled.

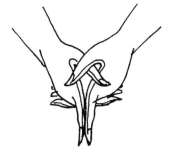

Ksepana
Two hands together in the gesture of 'sprinkling', i.e., the nectar of immortality.

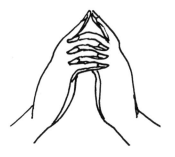

Uttarabodhi
Two hands placed together above the head with the index fingers together and the other fingers intertwined; the gesture of supreme enlightenment.

Asanas

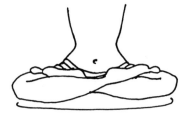

Padmasana
Also: vajrasana or dhyana asana. The well-known lotus position. There are a number of variations of this attitude in which the feet are placed in different positions.

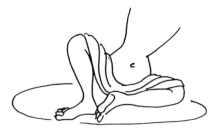

Lila asana
Sitting at ease. The right knee is pointing upwards and the right arm usually hangs loosely over the knee.

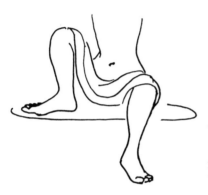

Rajalila asana
The king's posture. In this position it is quite clear that the figure is sitting on a throne: the left leg hangs down from the throne.

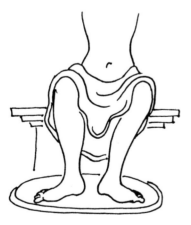

Bhadrasana
The 'Western' position. The feet are placed next to each other on the ground below. This position shows that the throne is not (yet) assured.

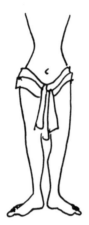

Samapada
The first of the standing asanas
with equal weight on both feet,
which are placed together.

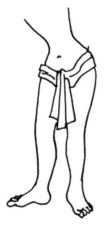

Tribhanga
The weight is on one leg; the
other leg is placed slightly for-
wards or to the side. The body is
bent at the hips and neck in
three separate parts.

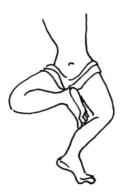

Chapastana

The arched position associated with flying. The leg carrying the weight with bended knee symbolizes the bow; the other leg, pulled up against the body, symbolizes the arrow.

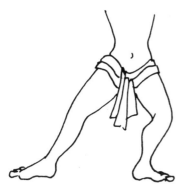

Alidha/pratyalidha

This position expresses the angry aspect of a deity. The left leg (alida) or right leg (pratyalida) is forcefully thrust to the side.

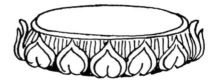

Padmasana
The lotus throne. When there is a double row of lotus leaves, it is known as 'visvapadmasana'. Sometimes this pedestal is also carried, e.g., by lions (singhasana), elephants (hatisana), a tortoise (kurmasana), or a mythical sea monster (makarasana).

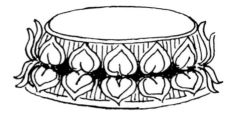

Ritual Attributes and Symbols

Daiji
Yin-yang. Original Chinese symbol of the two-in-one, especially of Samsara (the cycle of rebirth) and Nirvana.

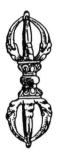

Vajra
Thunderbolt or (diamond) sceptre. Originally the symbol of the Vedic god Indra. Buddhist symbol of the imperturbable male principle that represents the path or method. The five points on each side symbolise the five Jinas (see p. 38). Tib: dorje.

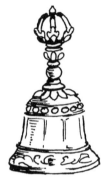

Ghanta
Bell. Symbolizes transience, the female principle that represents wisdom, the purpose. Together with vajra the symbol that leads to enlightenment, 'path and purpose are one'.

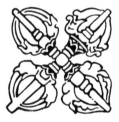

Visvavajra
Double vajra. Symbol of the conclusion of all actions, of the Absolute which is present in every direction.

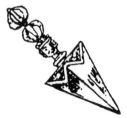

Vajrakila
Thunder nail; magical dagger. Serves to subordinate demonic counter-forces to the Doctrine, and literally 'nail them to the ground'. Symbol of insight breaking through.
Tib: phurbhu.

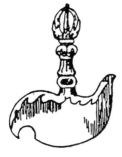

Kartika
Hatchet. Symbolizes the disintegration of all matter and all worldly bonds and their transformation into a positive force. Used in the Tibetan 'air burial'.

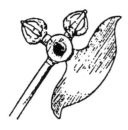

Parasu
Battle axe. Symbolizes the severance of all worldly attachments.

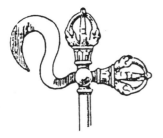

Ankusha
Stick for prodding elephants on their way. The hook with which those who doubt the doctrine of Buddha can be symbolically 'pulled'.

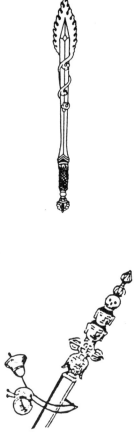

Khadga
Flaming sword. Destroyer of all ignorance and therefore a symbol of enlightenment.

Khatvanga
Magical staff; symbol of supernatural gifts (siddhi). There is always a row of skulls between the staff, which is made of wood, metal or bone, and the top (vajra, trisula or kapala).

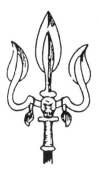

Trisula
Trident; weapon and symbol of Shiva. In Buddhism it is a symbol of Triratna, the Threefold Jewel: Buddha, Dharma and Sangha (see p. xiv and p. 25).

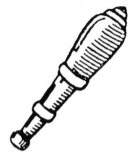

Gada
A staff with a tapering end used as a weapon in close combat. Also a symbol of office.

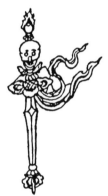

Danda
Sceptre staff; symbol of dominance. Similar to gada, but has a vajra or skull, possibly with ratna, as the knob.

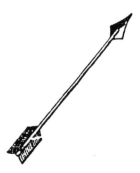

Shara
Arrow; The symbol of alertness and consciousness.

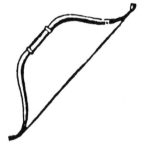

Chapa
Bow; together with the arrow, this is the symbol of the path and the purpose, method and wisdom, also of accurate determination.

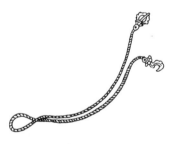

Pasha
Rope; this is used for catching demons and pulling those who have been removed from Dharma closer.

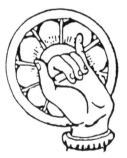

Khetaka
Shield; symbol of Dharma, the doctrine which protects like a shield.

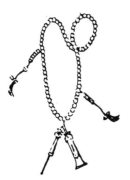

Akshamala
Rosary consisting of 108 beads. An invocation or mantra is said for every bead. Two separate strings of beads serve as a way of counting the number of 'rounds'.

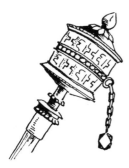

Prayer wheel
Devotional instrument. It contains the mantra OM MANI PADME HUM, written many times on a scroll of paper. The mantra becomes active every time the instrument is rotated.

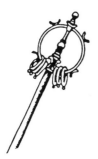

Khakkhara
Rattle staff; used by travelling monks to announce their arrival.

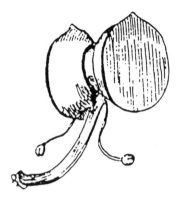

Damaru
Small drum; two half skulls with an animal's skin stretched over them. The sand-glass shape is made with a leather thong, with wooden beads at the end of the thong to make a rattling sound.

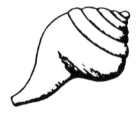

Sankha
Conch; the sound announces the glory of the holy name. The Tibetan conch trumpet has a richly carved metal setting with a mouthpiece.

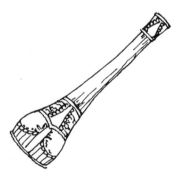

Kangling
Trumpet made from a human thighbone. The sound drives off evil spirits.

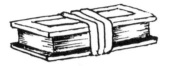

Pustaka
Book; the symbol of transcendental wisdom, and in particular, of the texts on the 'Perfection of Insight', the Prajnaparamita.

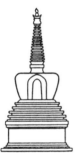

Stupa
Symbolic grave monument; originally the place where the ashes of a holy monk were kept. Now, especially the symbol of the Buddhist universe. The shape symbolizes the structure of the cosmos. Tib.: chörten.

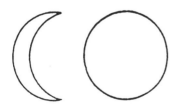

Chandra
Moon sickle or disc. Symbol of the unity of opposites.

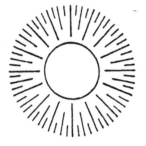

Surya
Sun; together with the moon, symbol of the unity in the apparent opposition between relative and absolute truth.

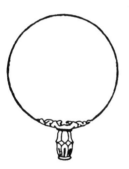

Adarsha
Mirror; symbol of the emptiness and lack of substance of the world.

Agni
Flame, fire; weapon of war and a common component in sacrifices.

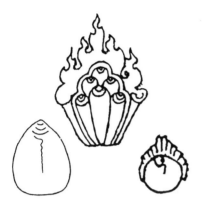

Ratna or Mani
Jewel. The representation of an oval stone, with or without a nimbus, symbolizes the 'Jewel of the Doctrine'. If the stone is a (small) round pearl with a nimbus, it is the magic jewel Cintamani, which fulfills every wish.

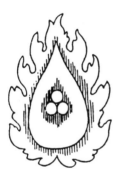

Triratna
The 'Three Jewels'; Buddha, Dharma and Sangha (see p. xiv).

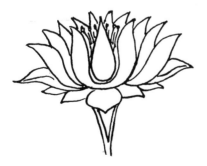

Padma
Open lotus flower, day lotus; can be any colour, except blue. Symbol of purity.

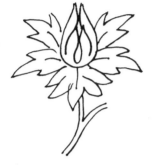

Utpala
Half-closed lotus flower, night lotus; in addition to purity, it represents the self-procreative and female principle. Nilotpala is the blue utpala.

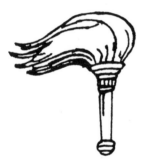

Chamara
Fly whisk made of yak hair; sign of dignity.

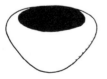

Patra
Begging bowl, especially of monks. When a seated figure holds a begging bowl on his lap, it means that he is the head of a monastic order.

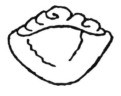

Kapala
Skull bowl; used in Tantric rituals for offering sacrificial meat or blood to protective deities to ensure their devotion.

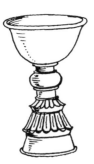

Dipa
Butter lamp; clarified butter (ghee) is burned in this as a sacrifice

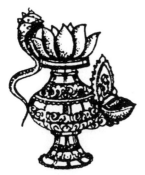

Sukunda
Oil lamp with its own oil reservoir, also used as a sacrificial lamp.

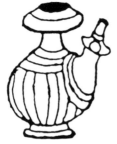

Bhumba
Sacrificial jug without a handle, intended for pouring water or nectar (in the hands of the one to whom the sacrifice is made). Also: Kamandalu.

Gau
Portable shrine in which a statue of the owner's personal deity (Ishtadevata) is kept wrapped in silk.

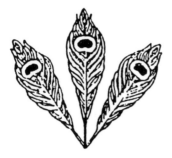

Mayurapattra
Peacock feathers; indicate an immunity to all poisons, i.e., all worldly temptations.

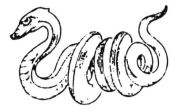

Naga
Snake; vestige of pre-Buddhist fertility rituals. Naga is still considered the god of rain, but also as the protector of Buddha's law.

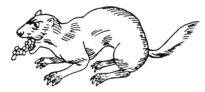

Nakula
Mongoose; keeper of all the jewels, who spews up all these riches when pinched by the god of wealth.

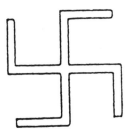

Swastika
Symbol of the law; sign of good fortune. It is one of the 65 signs of buddhahood which can be seen in Buddha's footprint.
Tib.: yung-drung.

The Ashtamangalas
(The 8 signs of good fortune)

The Ashtamangalas are often depicted either individually or together; together they are often shown as 'purna kalasha', a vase filled with all the characteristics of goodness. The Ashtamangalas are the attributes of *Ashtamangaladevi*, the goddess of good fortune (see p. 81).

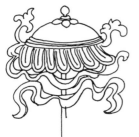

Chattra
Parasol; protection against all evil; high rank.

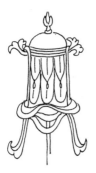

Dhvaja
Banner; the victory of Buddha's teachings.

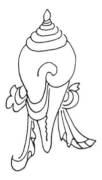

Sankha
Conch; absence of all evil, the
glory of holy men.

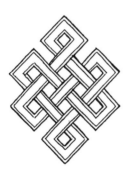

Shrivasta
An infinite knot; long life and
neverending love.

Dharmachakra
The Wheel of the Law; the eight
spokes represent the eightfold
path. Completion and salvation
through Buddha's teachings.

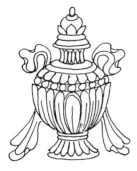

Kalasha
The vase of abundance; contains the water of immortality. Spiritual wealth.

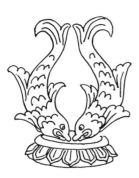

Matsyayugma
Golden fish; salvation from suffering, fertility.

Padma
The perfect lotus; purity.

Part 2

The Buddhas

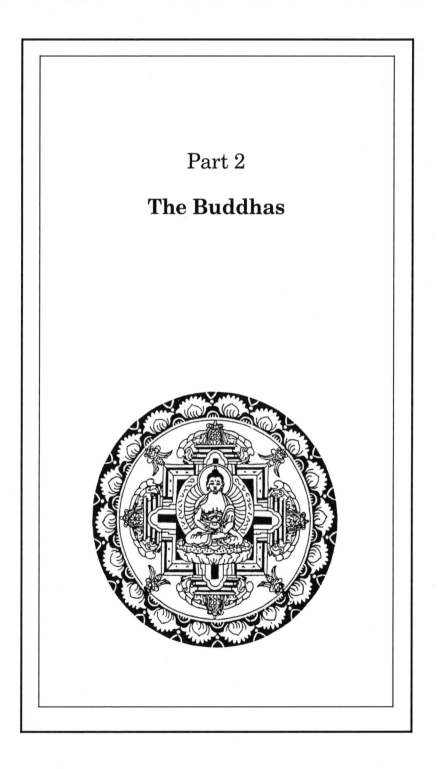

Manushi Buddhas

The term 'Buddha' refers to a being who has attained enlightenment and has been freed from the cycle of rebirth through his own insight. Thus there is not one Buddha, there are many. Most appear as manifestations of the Eternal Absolute, which is beyond time. These "transcendental Buddhas" are also lords over the various intermediary paradises. There, beings which have attained a particular level in their development towards enlightenment can be reborn to continue their development in complete tranquillity. But there are also manifestations which appear in the temporal world, and which have been incarnated or will be incarnated to show others the way to deliverance (Manushi Buddhas). They do not do this by intervening in the lives of their followers as a saviour. They merely act as teachers who lay down the Law (Dharma), show the way, and serve as an example for anyone who is prepared to follow the path. The historical *Buddha Gautama* was born in the 6th century BC as Prince Siddhartha, from the right side of his mother, Mayadevi. He was protected from the world by his father, King Suddhodana of the Shakya clan, who was afraid of what was to happen anyway: Siddhartha discovered the suffering in the world and decided to live a life of meditation. Fasting for long periods of time and self castigation did not bring him enlightenment; finally Gautama sat down under a tree and decided to stay there until he found the cause of suffering in the world. He eventually attained enlightenment under this bodhi tree. He died at the age of 80 (also see Introduction, pp. xiii, xiv and xv).

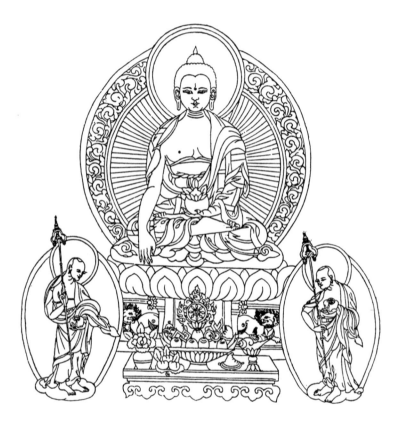

Buddha on the lion's throne.

Dipankara

Buddha Gautama himself declared that before him there had been other 'human Buddhas'. He mentioned six by name. These Buddhas have the same external features as Gautama: a top knot (ushnisa), a mark on the forehead (urna), and long earlobes. They can be identified by the different positions of their hands.

Dipankara, who is shown here, is considered to be the one who first brought the light (the Teachings) to the world. The six names mentioned by Gautama are: Vipasyin, Sikhin, Visvabhuja, Krakucchanda, Kanakamuni and Kasyapa.

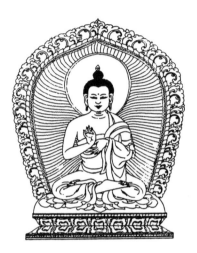

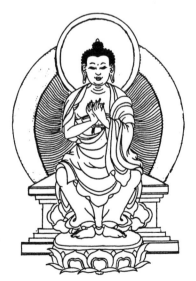

Maitreya

The future Buddha who will only reveal the teachings to the world again five thousand years after Gautama. Thus he is still a vision of the future, and that is why he is seated in the bhadrasana (p. 11). *Maitreya* will spend the time until he appears on earth as the Bodhisattva Natha in the heaven of the gods.

Transcendental Buddhas

Beyond time and natural laws, there are five transcendental Buddhas, the five abstract aspects of buddhahood. They are also called Jinas (conquerors), Tathagatas (the Perfect Ones) or Dhyani Buddhas (Meditation Buddhas).

These five incarnated forms of mystical wisdom have been placed in a detailed system over the course of the centuries, in which they each represent a family with related aspects and directions. In this way they demonstrate how the five skandas (aspects of the personality: body, experience, perception, spiritual stimulation, and consciousness) can be transformed. The two following pages give a summary of this system.

The illustration below shows the five Jinas with their Tantric partners in the yuganaddha position (Tib.: yab-yum). In every illustration in which it is depicted, this sexual embrace is the symbol of the total unification of opposites, of static wisdom with creative energy (the path and the object are one).

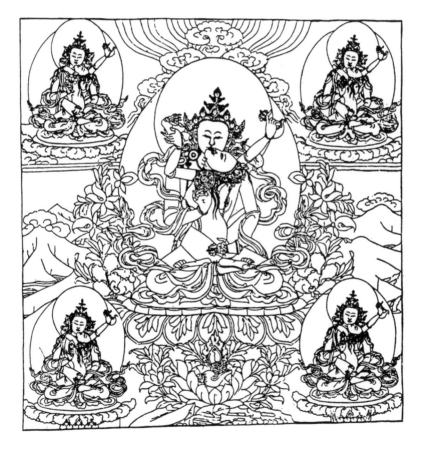

	Vairocana	**Akshobhya**
direction	centre	east
bija (mystical syllable)	OM	HUM
mudra	dharmachakra	bhumisparsa
meaning of the name	Illustrious	Imperturbable
family	Tathagata	Vajra
symbol	dharmachakra	vajra
colour	white	blue
skanda	vijnana	rupa
aspect of the personality	consciousness	form
negative energy	spiritual blindness	rage
wisdom	universal truth	neutral perception
element	ether	water
vaha (vehicle)	lion or dragon	elephant
prajna (partner)	Vajradhatvisvari	Locana
Bodhisattva (spiritual son)	Samanthabhadra	Vajrapani
Dakini	Buddha-dakini	Vajra-dakini

Ratnasambhava	Amitabha	Amogasiddhi
south	west	north
TRAM	HRIH	AH
varada	dhyana	abhaya
Born from a jewel	Boundless Light	Infallible success
Ratna	Padma	Karma
ratna	padma	visvavajara
yellow	red	green
vedana	samjna	samskara
experience	discernment	confirmation
arrogance	passion	envy
equality	insight	completion
earth	fire	air
horse or lion	peacock	harpy (Garuda)
Mamaki	Pandara	Syamatara
Ratnapani	Avalokiteshvara	Visvapani
Ratna-dakini	Padma-dakini	Visvavajra-dakini

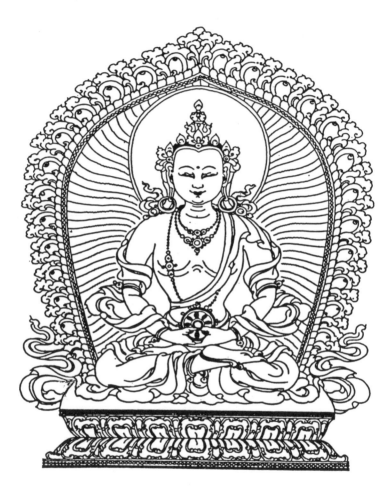

Vairocana

The lord of the centre, is seen as the combination of all the other Jinas, the "father". He is often depicted with four faces, so that he can see in every direction, and is omniscient. He is the incarnation of universal truth, Dharma.

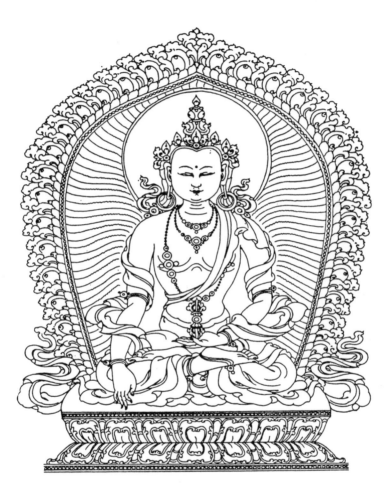

Akshobhya

The lord of the east, is the eternally imperturbable. In this illustration he is wearing the five-pointed crown which is often seen on the Jinas as a sign of the fact that they stand above all the laws of nature and transience.

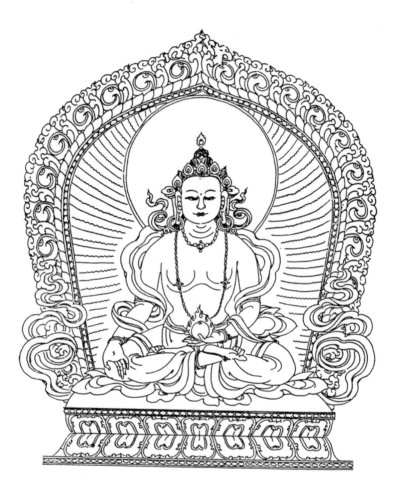

Ratnasambhava

The lord of the south, is the personification of generosity. In his hands he holds Cintamani, the jewel which fulfills every wish. But he does not only fulfill material needs; above all, he bestows love on all that is living.

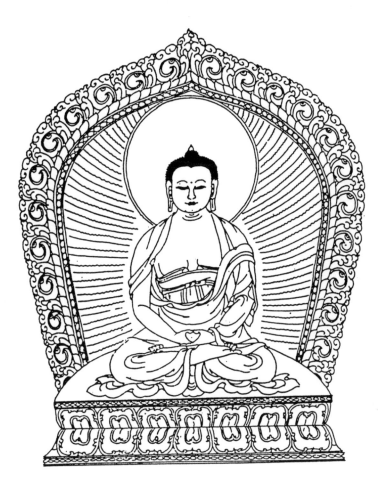

Amitabha

The lord of the west, is the oldest of the Jinas from a historical point of view, and the one who is most venerated. He is the incarnation of intuitive consciousness.

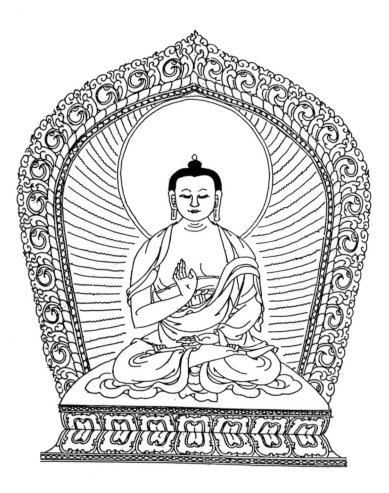

Amogasiddhi

The lord of the north, is the incarnation of the Buddha's 'practical wisdom', the wisdom which completes all workmanship. In his left hand he sometimes holds a visvavajra or a sword.

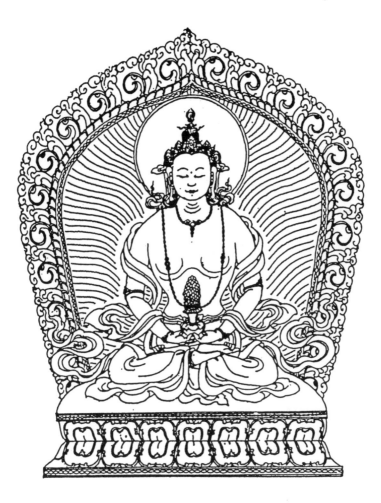

Amitayus

As the lord over the intermediary paradise, Sukhavati, Amitabha is
sometimes known as *Amitayus*. Thus, although they are actually the
same entity, Amitayus is also depicted differently. Instead of holding a begging bowl, he has a vase with the nectar of immortality in
his lap. The dark red colour of Amitabha is light red in Amitayus.

Adibuddha

In Mahayana Buddhism the idea evolved, probably inspired by the monotheism of Islam, that ultimately there is only one absolute power which creates itself, with no beginning and no end (Swayambhu). Originally this One Absolute manifests itself in the form of a flame springing from the heart of a lotus, but over the course of time this symbol was also personified in the form of the Adibuddha or Primordial Buddha. Vairocana is sometimes seen as Adibuddha, but there are other names and manifestations in which this supreme essence of buddhahood is presented, such as *Vajradhara*, shown below.

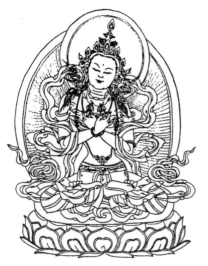

Vajradhara
The vajrahumkaramudra (the position of the hands with vajra and ghanta) is symbolic for the beatitude of the One, which results from the unity of opposites: the Unio Mystica.

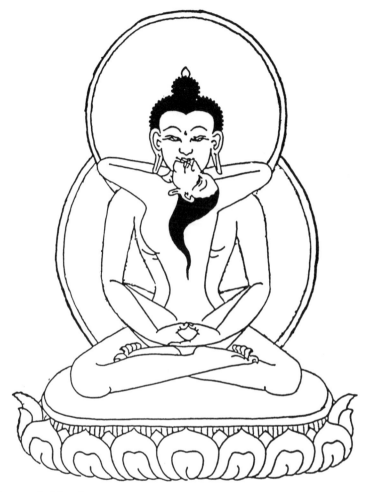

Samantabhadra
His name means Complete God. This manifestation of Adibuddha
(not to be confused with the Bodhisattva Samantabhadra) is shown
without any garments or attributes to demonstrate the fact that he
is totally himself. He is almost always accompanied by his prajna,
Samantabhadri, who is also completely naked. This Unio Mystica
shows how all beings, such as Samantabhadri, are derived from the
Absolute, but will ultimately be unified again when they have
shaken off all worldly bonds (symbolized here by the absence of
garments and attributes).

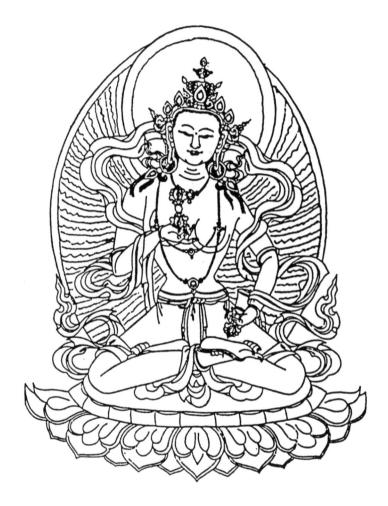

Vajrasattva

The Adibuddha Vajrasattva is sometimes considered as the sixth
Dhyani Buddha and as the high priest of the other five (particularly
in Nepal).

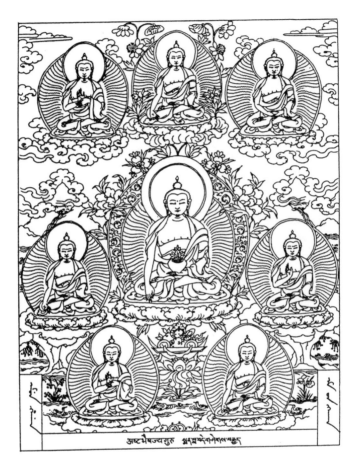

अष्टभेषज्यगुरु श्वरत्न्रोगोहगत्र्यश्रुद

The Buddhas of Medicine

The historical Buddha Gautama often called himself the healer of suffering in the world, and explained that Dharma was the medicine. This led to the idea that Gautama can be invoked in case of a disease to reveal the correct healing method to both the doctor and the sick person. In this function he is surrounded by seven healing aspects (see illustration), of which Bhaisajyaguru ('the Master of Healing' with the medicinal herb myrobalan, bearing a fruit with five lobes) is the only one who is sometimes depicted separately.

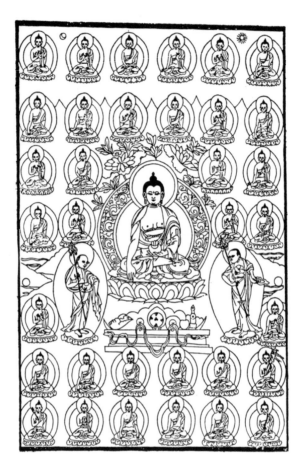

The 35 Buddhas of Purification

According to Indian tradition, there are 35 important violations of
Buddhist ethics.

However, there is a Buddha for every violation who will offer a
method for dealing with this obstacle on the path to enlightenment.
The Buddha will not give any practical help in this respect; he will
merely show the way. This also is one of the great differences between the Buddhas and the Bodhisattvas (see next chapter).

Part 3

The Bodhisattvas

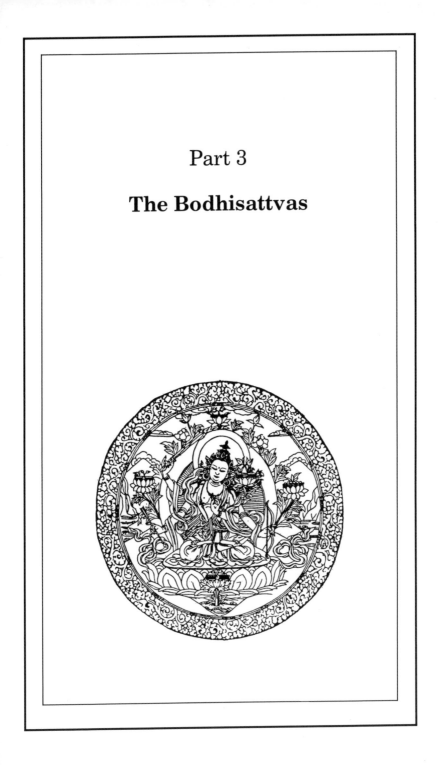

Bodhisattvas

A Bodhisattva is a being who has partly or completely attained the state of enlightenment. Buddha Gautama called himself a bodhisattva, a searcher for enlightenment, before he attained buddhahood. It is important for a bodhisattva that he not only pursues enlightenment for himself, but also for all other living creatures, and that he helps them in this.

There are ten stages (bhumi) in the bodhisattva's spiritual development. An elementary virtue (paramita) develops at every stage. In the seventh stage the bodhisattva becomes transcendent or Mahasattva. A Mahasattva, or Transcendental Bodhisattva, is a being that has achieved deliverance from the cycle of rebirth, but is postponing his ultimate, total redemption. Compassion (karuna) with all other beings leads the Mahasattva to remain voluntarily in the existing world to pursue the redemption of all beings. Because of his own pure state, the Mahasattva can destroy the burden of the karma of others. The Transcendental Bodhisattvas are no longer subject to the forces of any natural laws. They are able to assume any form they wish, to be in several places at once, and to move about at the speed of thought. The Bodhisattvas are considered to be the spiritual children of the abstract, and in that sense, unattainable, Dhyani Buddhas. They fulfil the role of intermediaries between Samsara (the existing world of illusion and suffering) and Nirvana (the state of calm, emotion-free bliss); and are at the same time the ideal of identification and the object of veneration.

The Mahasattva, who is probably the most popular and certainly the one of whom there are the most representations, is Avalokitesvara (the Lord who looks down). In Nepal there are 108 manifestations known of him. In Tibet, every rotation of the prayer wheel (see p. 21), every murmured mantra (Om Mani Padme Hum) is devoted to Avalokitesvara as the saviour in distress and redeemer of burdensome karma. When he appear as Lokesvara, he is sometimes considered to be derived from the Hindu god, Shiva.

After Avalokitesvara , the most popular Bodhisattva is Manjusri.

Avalokitesvara

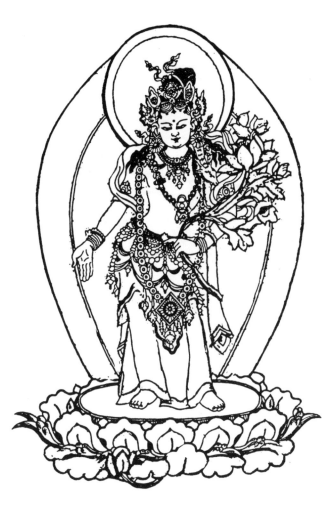

Padmapani

Of all the manifestations of Avalokitesvara, *Padmapani* is probably the oldest. He is the helper in cases of dire need, and the one who can shorten the path to deliverance from suffering. He can be recognized by his standing position (tribhanga). He wears the five-pointed crown of the conqueror of the world on his head, and the skin of a gazelle, the characteristic sign of Avalokitesvara, over his shoulder.

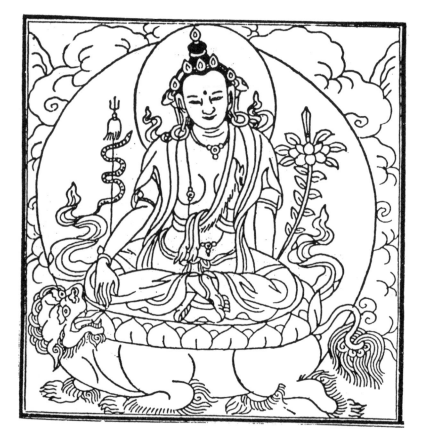

Simhanada-Lokesvara

The healer of all ills. His name and the animal on which he is mounted indicate this; there is a legend about a lion (simha) which brings back a stillborn cub to life with his roaring. Simhanada means 'the One with the lion's voice'. He is the healer who brings life back to the sick. His appearance is clearly similar to that of the Hindu god, Shiva: the top knot, sometimes with a crescent moon in it, the third eye, the trident, and the snake.

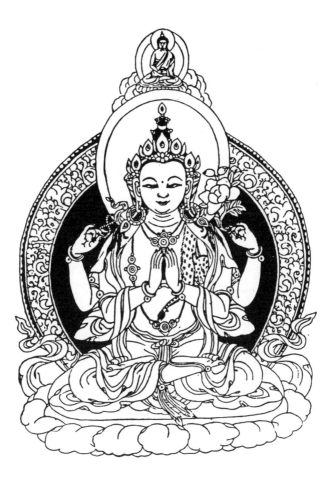

Sadaksari-Lokesvara

Also known as Kharchheri, is 'the Lord of the Six Syllables'. These six syllables belong to the mantra 'Om Mani Padme Hum', the expression of the deepest essence of Avalokitesvara. Sadaksari has four arms. In one hand he holds the akshamala (see p. 21), which serves to count the number of times that the mantra is spoken; in the other hand, he holds the lotus of absolute purity. He holds the magic jewel Cintamani in front of his chest (see p. 25). His spiritual father, Amitabha, is seated above his head.

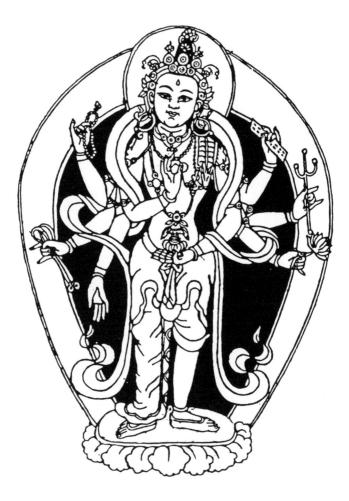

Amoghapasha-Lokesvara

'Lokesvara with the infallible rope', is a manifestation of Avalokitesvara as the Bringer of Truth and Deliverance, who has eight
arms. All his gestures and attributes relate to the proclamation of
the redeeming wisdom and the deterring of opponents (see p. 101).

Ekadasha-mahakarunika-Lokesvara is also known as Saman-thamukha, the All-sided. According to legend, Ekadasha descended from all-embracing compassion (mahakarunika) into hell and took a number of the inhabitants to the intermediate paradise, Sukhavati, only to discover that for every soul that was saved, a new soul was damned in hell.

His head broke into ten pieces with sorrow and dismay about the evil in the world. His spiritual father, Amitabha, made a new head from every piece and placed it on his son's trunk: nine faces full of love, one demonic face to help ward off evil more effectively, and at the top, Amitahba's own face. Each layer of three heads indicates that Ekadasha is looking at three worlds: the world of desire, the world of living forms, and the world without form.

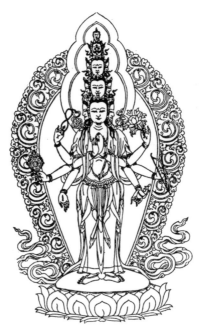

Sahasrabhuja-Lokesvara, 'the One with the thousand arms', like Ekadasha, has eleven heads, but in order to ensure that no creature goes without his all-embracing compassion, he has a thousand hands with an eye in the palm of every hand. In this way he is perfectly equipped to see all and intervene in everything. The thousand arms are depicted as a nimbus surrounding him.

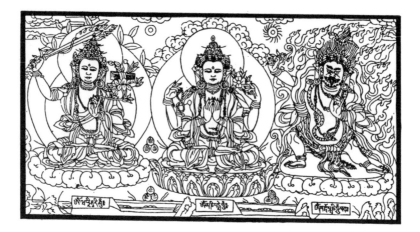

From left to right: Manjusri, Avalokitesvara, and the rain god Vajrapani: wisdom, compassion and protection against evil spirits.

Manjusri

He is sometimes considered to be the oldest Bodhisattva. There are various legends about him. In Nepal he is viewed as the founder of Nepalese culture; according to a Chinese legend he was created by Gautama himself and spread his Teachings in China; in Tibet he is praised every morning for banishing darkness once again. He is the Lord of Wisdom, who gives inspiration to everyone who wants to spread the teachings of Buddha. He is the Celestial Architect who shows how to build a worthy temple on earth.

Manjusri appears as the eternally youthful crowned prince of buddhahood in the form of *Arapacana.* In his right hand (the male side) he holds the flaming sword that destroys ignorance; in his left hand (the female side) he holds the book of transcendental wisdom, usually on a lotus flower.

As *Caturbhuja* who has four arms, Manjusri is holding a bow and arrow as a symbol of the accuracy of speech and philosophy.

As *Namasangiti* who has twelve arms, Manjusri makes the rather rare gesture of supreme enlightenment (uttarabodhimudra) with his hands joined together above his head.

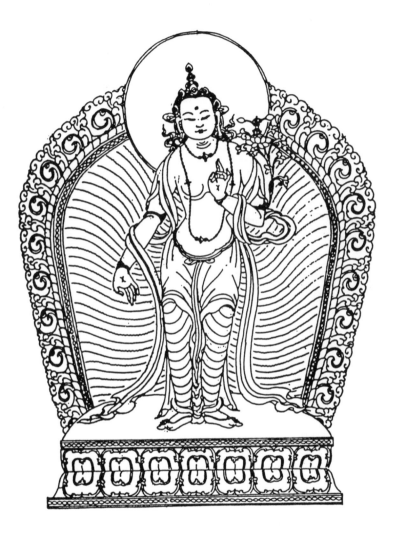

Vajrapani
Often depicted as Buddha's companion. On these occasions he is usually shown on the left while Padmapani is generally shown on the right. His origin lies in the Vedic god Indra (preceding Hinduism).
Some old representations show him as a muscular man with a beard.

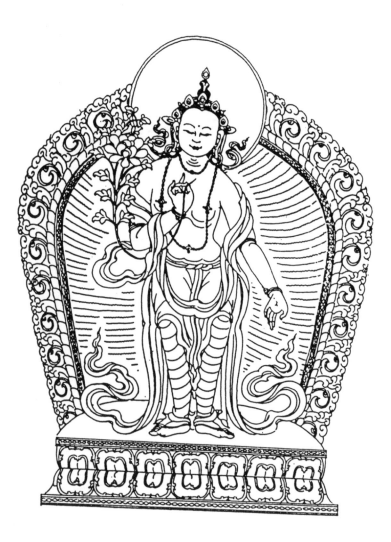

Samantabhadra

Often depicted together with Manjushri. His name means 'He who is most Blessed'. He can be easily distinguished from the Adibuddha Samantabhadra (see p. 49), because, in contrast with this Primordial Buddha, he is dressed and crowned.

Tara

In addition to the male Bodhisattvas there are also a number of female ones. *Tara* (Tib.:Drölma) is the most important of these. She represents the maternal aspect of compassion. Her name is related to the term 'cross over'; she protects people as they are crossing the 'Ocean of Existence'. According to legend, she was created from a tear of Avalokitesvara.

Tara appears in 21 different forms in various colours, of which the White and Green are the oldest. These two Taras are historically related to the two wives of King Srongtsen Gampo, who brought Buddhism to Tibet from Nepal and China respectively (see p. 88).

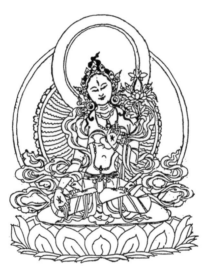

White Tara (Sitatara or Svetatara) can easily be recognized by the seven eyes in her head, the palms of her hands and the soles of her feet. In this way she can perceive anyone who needs her help in any direction.

She is usually holding an open white lotus as a symbol of her purity.

Green Tara (Syamatara or Harit Tara) is seen as the protector against all dangers.

Her colour is green. The lotus in her hand is blue and half open (nilotpala). Sometimes there are two lotuses. She does not have any extra eyes (see p. 66).

Green Tara

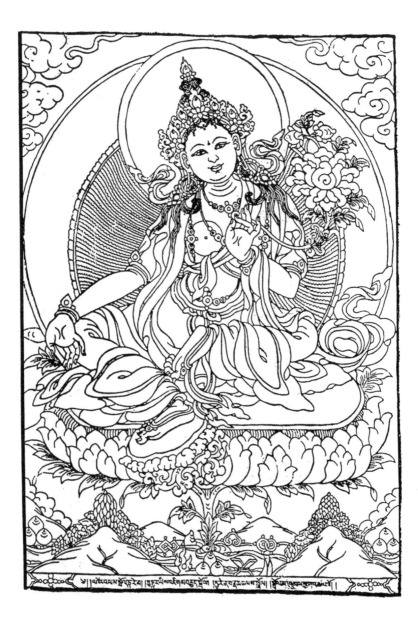

Part 4

Deities

and

Divine Beings

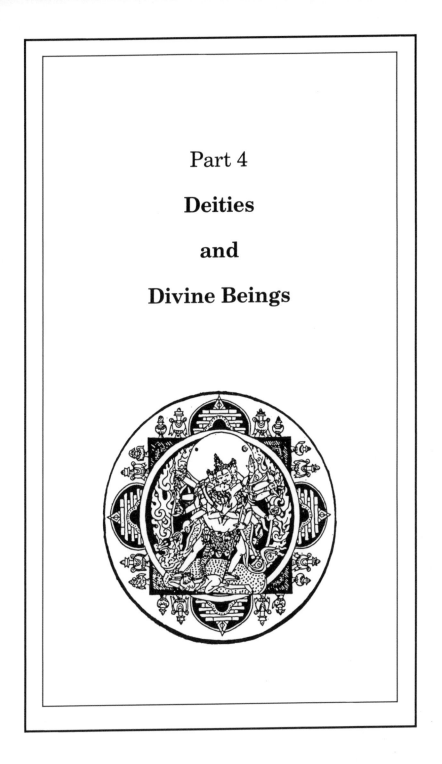

Yidams

The teachings of the Tantric path to enlightenment can be found in a number of texts which contain so much secret knowledge that they can only be understood after years of study and with the help of a teacher who has been initiated. For this reason the Tantric principle of the path to enlightenment which leads through all human experience has been given a more easily recognizable form in the Ishtadevatas (the personal or inner gods), or *Yidams*, as they are known in Tibet.

In order to attain the serenity of a Buddha, a Sadhaka (pupil of Tantra) must learn to conquer many different inner obstacles. A Yidam confronts the Sadhaka with his own weaknesses and gives him the inner strength to conquer his fear to achieve true self knowledge, and to transform his 'faults' into wisdom which will lead to redemption.

In most cases the Yidams are depicted in an ecstatic embrace with their Yogini, an ecstasy which greatly transcends self-interest and passion. All the bonds with the world of illusion are broken.

As the Tantra itself is full of secret doctrines, the meaning of its visible symbols is not easy to indicate. Nevertheless, Heruka is probably the most representative manifestation of Yidam. He has eight faces, sixteen arms and four legs. He is seen as the destroyer of all Maras (the demon of illusion and temptation, and his helpers). Usually he is depicted embracing his female partner, Nairatma, to symbolise the removal of all contrasts, which brings about a blissful unity. In this form the Yidam is called *Hevajra*.

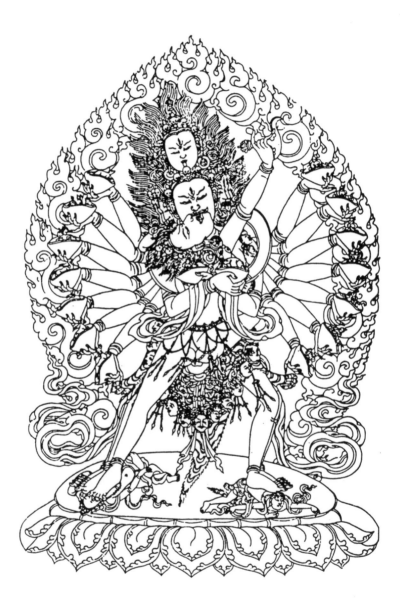

Hevajra

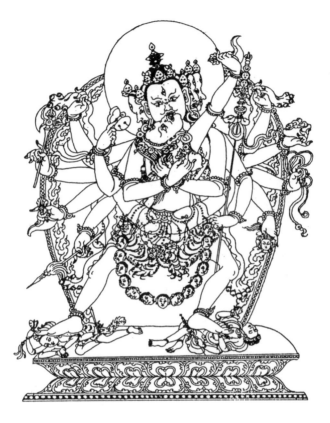

Sambara

Also called Samvara, known in full as Chakrasamvara. Is always depicted with the Yogini, Vajravarahi. This Dakini, who can be identified by the pig's head on the side of her head, is herself a Yidam. Together they represent the supreme beatitude which resides in the removal of duality. Sambara usually has four heads and twelve arms.

Apart from the Yidams depicted here, there are many others. Two of the most important are:
Kalachakra, the personification of a Tantra who uses astrology; he has four heads and twelve or twenty-four arms; and *Vajrabhairava*, who is both a Yidam and one of the Dharmapalas (see p. 73). One of his functions is to keep all the uninitiated away from the great Tantric mysteries.

Gods and Goddesses

Buddhism has spread in many countries and cultures, always integrating the local gods into the system.

For example, there are Hindu gods, Bön gods (the ancient religion of Tibet) and local gods in Mahayana and Tantrayana Buddhism.

In order to place this entire pantheon correctly within the Buddhist teachings of karma (the meaning of acts in the light of the purpose of enlightenment) and redemption, the gods are classified amongst the beings which have not yet been delivered from the cycle of rebirth but who have acquired a great deal of positive karma.

Therefore it is best to consider a deity as a function (such as the gift of fertility, health, protection against demons, etc.) which is always performed by a supernatural being (deva) which has not yet been redeemed. This being must give up his function when he has used all his good karma and another deva will take over that function. There are peaceful gods and goddesses (Shanta) and terrible ones (Krodha).

Manjusri (p. 62)   *Avalokitesvara (p. 57)*   *Vajrapani (p. 77)*

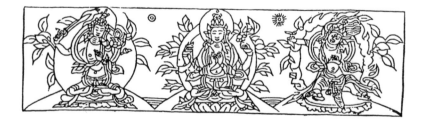

The Eight Dharmapalas

The eight Dharmapalas were originally hostile demons but they were tamed by Padmasambava (see p. 89) by means of his magical strength and now act as the fiery defenders of Dharma (the Teachings). They are also viewed as wrathful manifestations of Bodhisattvas, who help the pupil to attain supreme insight. For this purpose they are often assembled in a special temple (Tib.: gonkhang). They are incarnations of the powers of dissolution and transformation, the powers which can bring about a breakthrough in meditation.

The Dharmapalas can be recognised by their red hair, flaming aureoles and crowns consisting of five skulls.

They are also known as the Ashtabhairava (the eight which inspire fear).

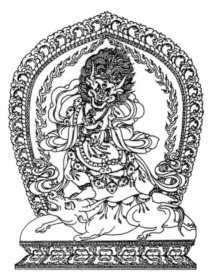

Yamantaka is the conqueror of the demon of death, Yama. He appears in different manifestations: with one head and a vajra in his hair (to distinguish him from his arch-enemy whom he resembles in this form), but also with 9 heads, 34 arms and 16 legs. In this case he is known as Vajrabhairava and is viewed as the wrathful manifestation of Manjusri.

In both forms he is also depicted with his female partner, the Yogini, Vidyadhara.

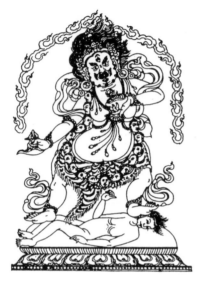

Yama

After being defeated by Yamantaka the god of death *Yama* himself became a Dharmapala. He decides to which realm of rebirth the dead will go, depending on their karma. In this respect he is so important that he has been given the honorary title of Dharmaraja (Dharma king). Like Yamantaka he is often seen with the head of a buffalo, though without a vajra. He can, even with a normal face, also be identified by the Dharmachakra (the Wheel of the Law) on his chest.

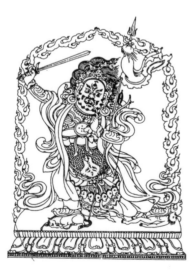

Beg-ts'e

Before he became a Dharmapala, *Beg-ts'e* was a Tibetan god of war. This is apparent from his name which also describes his appearance: "One with armour under his garments".

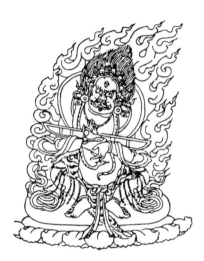

Mahakala

A Dharmapala who appears in many different forms. A number of these are derived from ancient Hindu and Tibetan gods; in his most important manifestation Mahakala ("the Great Black One") is a Buddhist form of the Hindu god Shiva. In many manifestations he is depicted with a trident (trisula) and a different number of arms. In other illustrations he has an object which sometimes looks like an official staff or a club but is considered by some to be a bundle of tent poles: Mahakala is the god who protects Mongolia and the tents of the nomads. Sometimes he is also accompanied by the celestial being Garuda, the bird man.

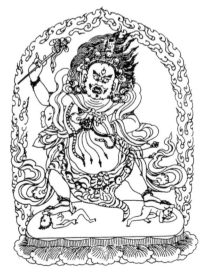

Hayagriva

The easiest to identify of all the Dharmapalas, viz. by the horse's head in his hair. He originated from Hinduism where he was one of the manifestations of Vishnu. In Buddhism he is sometimes viewed as an incarnation of the Dhyani Buddhas Amithaba or Aksobhya.

Hayagriva is the guardian of the sacred texts who scares his enemies away with his whinnying.

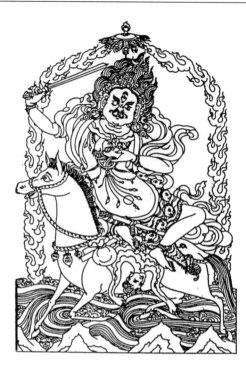

Devi Lhamo

She is the only female Dharmapala and perhaps the most fearful.
She is the Buddhist form of the Hindu goddess Kali, the goddess of
destruction. Lhamo brings death and destruction to the opponents of
Dharma. She appears in different forms but is usually depicted with
a crown of heads, a human skin wrapped around her shoulders, the
sun in her navel and the moon in her hair, riding a white donkey.
The reins are poisonous snakes, a bag of diseases hangs from the
saddle and in her hand she holds a skull full of blood. In addition she
is often accompanied by two terrible natural spirits, so-called Yakshas.

The two Dharmapalas *Sitabrahman* and *Kubera* are not illustrated
here. They are the only two who are not represented with a crown of
skulls and their faces are not demonic although they are grim. Sitabrahman (the 'White Brahman') can be identified by his sleeved
tunic and the turban on his head. Kubera is a manifestation of Jambhala who can be distinguished from Jambhala by his flaming
aureole (see p. 80).

In addition to the Dharmapalas there are a number of gods who closely resemble them but do not have the function of protecting the Dharma. These are mainly integrated Hindu gods with a specialist "field" who are known as "Krodha gods" just as the Dharmapalas.

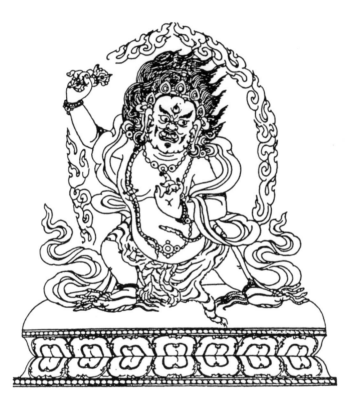

Vajrapani
In Buddhism there are two totally different entities derived from the Vedic god of rain and thunder, Indra. These both have the same name. One is the Bodhisattva Vajrapani, the other is Vajrapani, the god of rain. The latter is often viewed as the guardian of the secret Tantric law.
He can be identified in particular by the snakes (Nagas) beneath his feet which are a symbol of water and fertility.

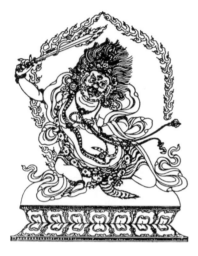

Acala

The vidyaraja ('king of the redeeming knowledge') *Acala* is considered in China and Japan as the advocate of the dead. When the deceased stands eye to eye with Yama, who weighs his karma, it is Acala who reveals his positive karma.

In Hinduism 'Acala' is another name for Shiva.

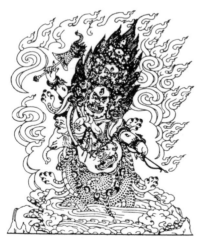

Rahu

The nine planets and their respective gods are known as the Navagrahas. *Rahu* is the Lord of them all.

His nine heads each represent a planet, including the sun and the moon. He wears his own head on his stomach. With his enormous mouth he swallows up the sun or the moon from time to time thus causing a solar or lunar eclipse.

The Four Digpalas

According to ancient views, the Guardians of the Four Directions the Lokapalas or Digpalas, are warriors who have the task of protecting Buddha against earthly threats.

Later on they acted in particular as guardians of the world against penetrating demons. In addition, each one is Lord over an army of mythical beings.

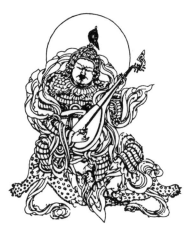

Dhritarastra, the guardian of the east is Lord over the Gandharvas, celestial musicians who float in the air.

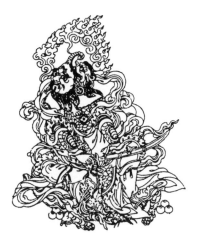

Virudhaka, the guardian of the south is Lord over the Kumbhandas, dwarves with the faces of buffalos.

In Nepal there is another view of the Digpalas which entails that they are the Guardians of Four Directions. Some of these are familiar from the Hindu pantheon.

The eight are: Indra, the king of the gods, east; Agni, god of fire, south east; Yama, god of death, south; Nairitya, god of fear, south west; Varuna, god of the ocean, west; Vayu, god of wind, north west; Kubera, god of wealth, north; Isana, a manifestation of Shiva, north east.

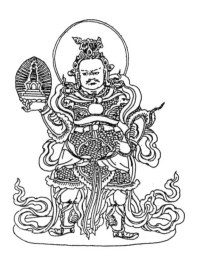

Virupaksa, the guardian of the west is also guardian of Buddhist relics. He is Lord of the Nagas: snakes.

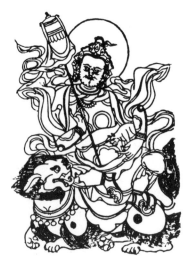

Jambhala, also known as Vaishravana or Kubera, is the guardian of the north but is also known as the separate god of wealth and prosperity. He is Lord of the Yakshas.

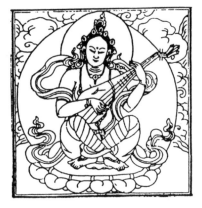

The goddess **Sarasvati** has moved directly from Hinduism into the Buddhist pantheon, without any change in her name or significant adaptations of her appearance. She is the goddess of the "audible arts": music, poetry and rhetoric.

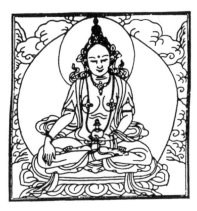

Vasundhara, like her Hindu counterpart Lakshmi, is the goddess of well being and has many worshipers. She grants everything that is needed for a life without hardship: piety and wisdom for a rich spiritual life, the Three Jewels and fertility in the fields for the fulfillment of worldly needs, a long life and her help and support for a physical existence without problems. She is sometimes depicted with one head, but often with three heads and six arms.

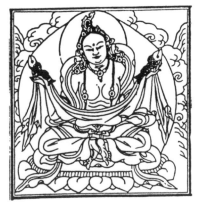

Ashtamangaladevi is the goddess of good fortune who is often depicted surrounded by the eight signs of good fortune (also see p. 30). Here she is shown only with the golden fish.

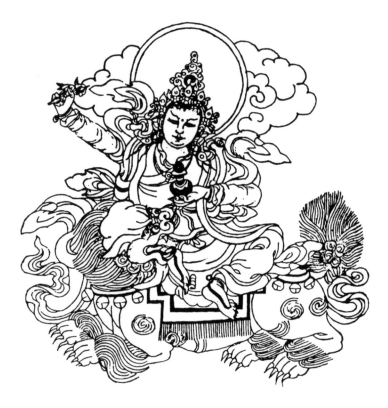

Travellers in the Himalayas, especially on the Tibetan side, always make sure they do not get in the way of the Five Sisters of Good Fortune. If these mountain nymphs are well disposed towards travellers, they will help and protect them on their journey but woe betide anyone who does not please them for any reason. Storms, icy cold weather, and accidents will probably befall him ... In addition to their involvement with travellers the five sisters of good fortune also have the task of protecting hermits who meditate in isolated caves high up in the mountains. They can be identified in particular by the animals on which they are mounted, seated with both legs to one side.

They are respectively *Sugati*, on a dragon; *Suganthi*, on a buck; *Sumukhi*, on a wild donkey; *Sumati*, on a tiger, and finally **Dirgha-yusi** (illustrated above) who is mounted on a lion.

Dakinis and Yoginis

In order to attain redemption and achieve insight into the secrets of the Tantric writings, it is also possible to appeal to the divine female intermediaries who are each said to have access to a Transcendental Buddha. In this way they can pass the insights of this Buddha to the seeker for deliverance. If her main task is to reveal demonic forces and chase them away the goddess concerned appears in her terrible form as a Dakini. If her intention is to mobilize the sexual power of the yogin (one who practices Tantra) in order to proceed towards enlightenment, she will appear as a seductive maiden, Yogini.

Whatever her appearance her attitude always expresses movement to show how she flies to fulfill her role as an intermediary between Buddha and the yogin and as a symbol of the specific intense energy which she represents.

The illustration on the next page shows the so called **Buddhadakini** who goes with the Jina of the centre: Vairocana, as an example of a Dakini who has access to one Dhyani Buddha. The other Jinas are accompanied respectively by the *Vajra-dakini* (Akshobhya), the *Ratna-dakini* (Ratnasambhava), the *Padma-dakini* (Amitabha), and the *Visvavajra-dakini* (Amogasiddhi).

The *Sarvabuddha-dakini* has access to all the Jinas. Her appearance is distinguished from the other Dakinis mainly by her wild hair and the skull full of blood which she holds. She is also sometimes called the Red Dakini.

Buddhadakini

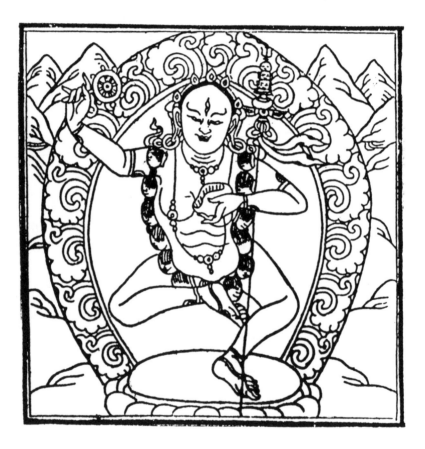

Part 5

Miscellaneous

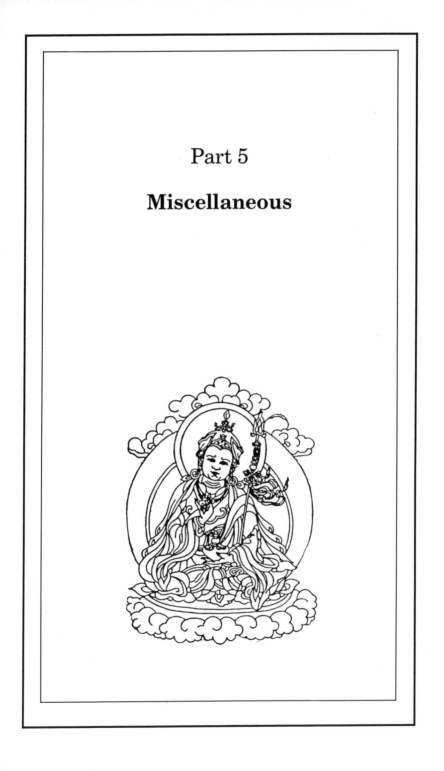

Human Beings

A number of people played an important role in the history of Mahayana Buddhism and Tantrayana Buddhism. There is a wealth of stories about gurus (teachers), arhats (holy men), siddhas (Tantric masters who have developed supernatural powers: siddhi and acaryas (learned monks who have made a mark on Buddhism by writing books or commentaries or founding a new order). These stories go back centuries to a distant past.

Of all the things that could be related about Buddha Gautama and the spread and development of different schools of Buddhism, we have chosen for the purpose of this book, to concentrate on the way Buddhism spread and developed in Tibet. Tibetan Lamaism has a special place in the practice of Tantric law and the expressions of the principles of that law. In addition, a number of gurus, arhats, siddhas and acaryas who played a role in this development have acquired fame which extends beyond the small circle of local followers.

The survey given below is not drawn up in any ritual order (see p. xi), but in a more chronological order which is easier for the layman to understand.

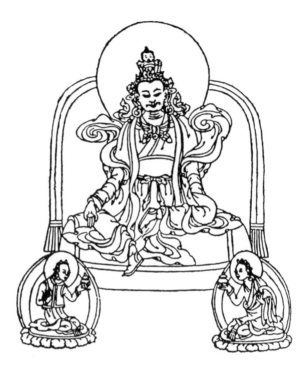

Srongtsen Gampo

Traditionally, the history of Buddhism started in Tibet with King *Srongtsen Gampo*. In the 7th century he founded the city of Lhasa and married two Buddhist princesses: the daughter of the Chinese emperor and the daughter of the King of Nepal. These royal brides brought the Buddhist Teachings with them and had the first small Buddhist shrines built.

Srongtsen Gampo is usually depicted sitting on a throne with his two wives kneeling before him. The head of Amitabha is on top of his crown.

Just over a century and four kings later, not much had survived of the Buddhist Teachings and the shrines founded by the two princesses. The priests of the ancient Bön religion were responsible for this.

King *Trhisong Detsen* changed this state of affairs for good. He rebuilt the temples which had fallen into ruin, and invited buddhist masters from India to come to Tibet. After his reign, Buddhism was always of central importance in Tibet.

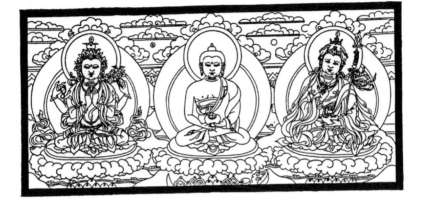

Padmasambhava

One of the men invited by Trhisong Detsen to restore Buddhism in Tibet was the Indian siddha *Padmasambhava*. He had a profound knowledge of the Tantra and had developed extraordinary supernatural gifts. Trhisong Detsen asked him to fight the demons (the gods of the Bön religion) and Padmasambhava did so with great success. One by one they were subordinated to his authority, and then he forced them to use their powers for the benefit of the Buddhist religion (also see Dharmapalas page 73). Many legends arose about Padmasambhava, his magical powers and his 25 lobmas (pupils). He is considered as the author of the Tibetan Book of the Dead (bardo thödol).

There are illustrations of Padmasambhava in different forms. One of the most common manifestations is a triptych which symbolises the Three Vehicles (see p. xiv). Buddha Gautama is seated in the middle as the personification of the doctrine of Hinayana with Avolokitesvara at his right hand as the personification of Mahayana, and Padmasambhava at his left hand (identified by the khatvanga and the hat with the raised ear-flaps) as the personification of Tantrayana (see illustration above).

Tilopa, Naropa and Marpa

The oldest known Buddhist guru is *Tilopa* (10th century). He lived in India and seems to have acquired his knowledge of the teachings not by studying under a guru but by his own exercises and experiments. He developed exceptional siddhi and gained great fame as Mahasiddha (great siddha).

Tilopa's best known pupil is *Naropa* (10th and 11th century). Naropa was an inspired speaker and had a gift for explaining mystical dreams and visions. His pupil *Marpa* (11th century) wrote down Naropa's teachings. Naropa is also known as "the Translator", because he translated the Indian Buddhist books as well as Naropa's teachings into Tibetan.

Tilopa, Naropa and Marpa were successively the first three heads of the Kagyu order, one of the four great orders of Tibetan Buddhism. The others are: Nyingma, Sakya and Gelug.

Milarepa

Marpa's most famous pupil was Mila (11th/12th century) who was later known as *Milarepa* or Mila-raspa (Mila with the cotton cloth). He became famous particularly for his strictly ascetic lifestyle and his poems "The Hundred Thousand Songs".

Milarepa is easy to recognise in illustrations: he holds his right hand behind his ear so as to hear more clearly the music of the spheres and the voice of the Teachings.

Milarepa's spiritual heir was *Gampopa* who developed the Kagyu order as a well organised institution.

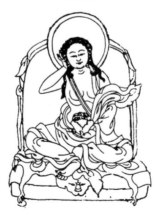

Tsongkapa

In the 14th century *Tsongkapa*, the reformer, founded a new order in Tibet. This was the order of the Gelugpas (the "virtuous") which revived the importance of celibacy. This order was also known as the order of the Yellow Hats. The Dalai Lama belongs to this order.

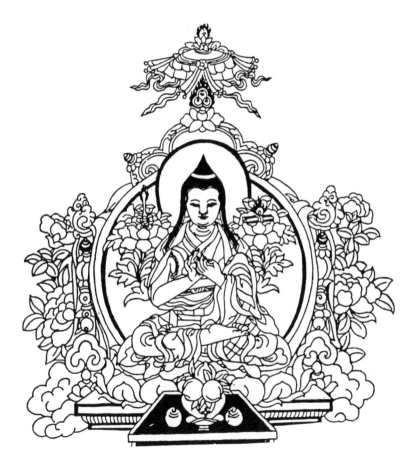

Ganesh

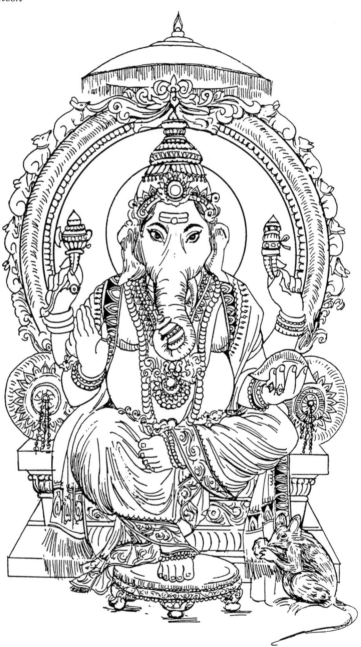

Hindu Gods

A number of the gods from the Vedas and the Hindu pantheons have been assimilated into Buddhism. Indra, Vishnu and Shiva have been mentioned several times. Sarasvati transferred directly (see p. 81); the bird man, Garuda, carries Vishnu, but we also see him in some illustrations of Amoghasiddhi and Mahakala. The god with the elephant head *Ganesh* has a very special place. This son of Shiva and Parvati is a true Hindu god but is also worshipped in Jainism and in Buddhism. In Hinduism he is the god of wisdom. He clears away all obstacles of any nature and is the protector of science, writing and schools.

In one of the manifestations of Mahakala the latter pushes a figure who can clearly be recognised as Ganesh against the ground. This is a way of saying that Mahakala, the Buddhist protector of wisdom, is mightier than the Hindu protector of wisdom, Ganesh. However, this form of rivalry is exceptional. For instance, the entrance of many Buddhist temples in the valley of Kathmandu in Nepal is guarded by the same Ganesh, who protects wisdom wherever it may be found, impartially, like a true god.

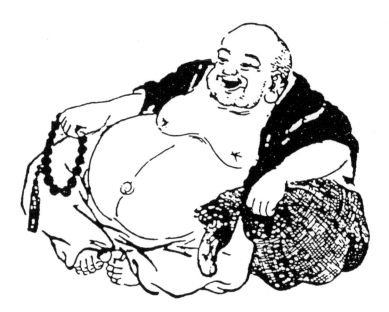

The Laughing Buddha

He can be found everywhere made of soapstone or gilt amongst the chop sticks, in markets even in our own western countries: a laughing figure with a bald head and a fat, bare stomach. This figure is known as the "Laughing Buddha". You will not have found him amongst the historical and transcendental Buddhas shown in this booklet, for the Laughing Buddha is not a manifestation of one of those Buddhas, as many people incorrectly imagine. "The Laughing Buddha" is another name for the Chinese master of Zen, Poe-Tai Ho-shang who lived between the 6th and 10th century and discovered 'the Buddha within himself'. He wandered through China without any cares and was perfectly happy, often surrounded by children. After his death he was worshipped as a popular hero and god of good fortune. In that function he is still wandering all over the world as a tangible expression of unconcerned beatitude which can be attained by anyone when he finds his own true nature, the 'Buddha within himself'.

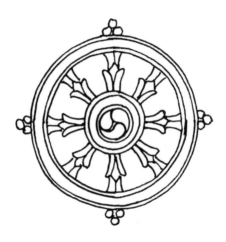

Appendix

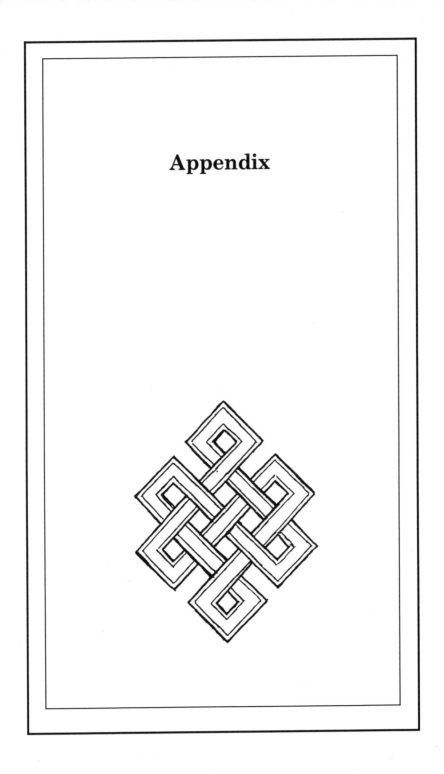

Aid to Identification

The multitude of different beings and their various manifestations means that it is often difficult to determine who is depicted in a statuette or picture of these figures. The list given below will help to identify them. It includes the most important categories and a number of figures.

BUDDHAS

Lotus position (except for Maitreya, and in some of the scenes from the life of Siddharta); short, close cropped frizzy hair; often covered with a five pointed crown in the Transcendental Buddhas.
Top knot with a jewel on top of it; stretched ear lobes; mark on the forehead.
The historical and Transcendental Buddhas are usually wearing monk's clothes; the latter may also be dressed in regal garments.

Gautama
Bhumisparsamudra, often with a begging bowl in the other hand; sometimes also dharmachakramudra. Often shown on the "lions throne".
Dipankara
Hands in front of his chest, right hand in vitarkamudra.
Maitreya
'Western' position on throne or standing.

Vairocana
White. Disc of the sun or Wheel of the Law in his lap. Sometimes has four faces.
Akshobya
Blue. Right hand in bhumisparsamudra. A vajra in his lap.
Ratnasambhava
Yellow. Right hand in varadamudra. Cintamani in his lap.
Amitabha
Red. Hands in dhyanamudra. With begging bowl: Lord of the intermediate paradise Sukhatvati.
Amoghasiddhi
Green. Right hand in abhayamudra, sometimes with visvavajra in his lap.
Amitayus
Dark red. Can also be distinguished from Amitabha by the bottle of nectar.
Vajradhara
Crown, hands in vajrahumkaramudra.
Samantabadhra
Completely naked without any attributes, in yab-yum.
Vajrasattva
Crown, vajra in front of his chest, ghanta in his lap.

BODHISATTVAS

Third eye or mark on forehead; peaceful facial expression; calm standing or sitting position; two legs. Usually one head, in some cases between three and eleven heads. Number of arms varies between 2 and 1,000.

Avalokitesvara. Skin of a gazelle over the shoulder.
Padmapani
Sweet appearance, many ornaments. Usually standing in tribangha, sometimes seated. Right hand in varadamudra, lotus flower in left hand.

Lokesvaras
Simhanada
Seated on a lion: has a trishula with a snake.
Sadaksari
Lotus position; Amitabha is seated above or over his head. Four arms. Attributes; prayer beads, lotus, Cintamani.
Amoghapasha
Standing. Eight arms; one right hand in vitarkamudra and one in varadamudra. Attributes: prayer beads, lasso, book, trident, lotus, vase.
Ekadasha-maharunika
Standing. Eleven heads, eight arms, one right hand in varadamudra. Attributes: prayer beads, wheel, lotus, bow and arrow, jug, Cintamani.
Sahasrabhuja
(Not illustrated). Same as Ekadasha – maharunika but with an 'aureole' of 'a thousand' arms. Sometimes there are actually a thousand, sometimes fewer.

Manjusri, always with a flaming sword and book.
Arapacana
Manjusri in his usual manifestation with two arms.
Caturbhuja
(Not illustrated). Four arms. Extra: bow and arrow.
Namasangiti
(Not illustrated). Twelve arms. Attributes the same as Caturbhuja plus the following mudras: dharmachakra, ksepana and uttarabodhi.

Tara, a woman in different colours.
White Tara
Eyes in the palms of her hands and soles of her feet; usually with a white open lotus.
Green Tara
Green, with blue half closed lotus, sometimes two lotus flowers.

GODS ETC.

Yidams
Third eye; grim facial expression. Often several faces and in yab-yum.

Dharmapalas
Third eye; flaming aureole. Five pointed crown (usually skulls); wild streaming red hair; demonic face; position of legs alida or pratya-lida. Kubera and Sitabrahman are exceptions to this. Other Krodha gods have similar characteristics.

Dakinis
Third eye, grim, 'witch-like' face. Often in arched position (cha-pastana); right hand often raised in karanamudra and left hand in front of the chest with elbow bending out to the side.

Yoginis
Appearance of beautiful young maiden. Often with flaming aureole. Sometimes in flying position.

Hatchet and skull bowL are 'common attributes for both dakinis and yoginis.

MISCELLANEOUS

Head of the order
Identified by the begging bowl in his lap.

Historical figures
Often looking to one side. Apart from uncovered heads with all sorts of human hairstyles, there are various head coverings including the mitra (pointed cap) with flaps which hang down or are turned up.

Bibliography

Short description of Gods, Goddesses and Ritual Objects of Buddhism and Hinduism in Nepal
Published by H.A.N., Kathmandu, Nepal

The Art of Nepal – Lydia Aran
Sahayogi Prakashan, Tripureshwar, Kathmandu, Nepal

Buddhistische Bilderwelt, Ein ikonographisches Handbuch des Mahayana und Tantrayana-Buddhismus – Hans Wolfgang Schumann
Eugen Diedrichs Verlag, Cologne

Tantra, yoga en meditatie, De Tibetaanse weg naar verlichting – Erik Bruijn
Published by Ankh-Hermes B.V., Deventer

Tibetan Thangka Painting, Methods and Materials – David & Janice Jackson
Snow Lion Publications, Ithaca, New York, USA

The Tibet Guide – Stephen Batchelor
Wisdom Publications, London 1987

Godenbeelden uit Tibet – Hugo Kreijger
SDU Uitgeverij, Openbaar Kunstbezit, Amsterdam 1989

Kunst aus dem Himalaya "Stutzen des Inneren", Katalog zur gleichnamigen Ausstellung – Dr. Andrea Loseries-Leick

Hinduism – Shakunthala Jagannathan
Vakils, Feffer & Simons, Bombay, India 1984

The Hindu Pantheon – Edward Moor, F.R.S.
J. Johnson, London 1810; Asian Educational Services, New Delhi 1981

PRANA no. 56, summer 1989
De Goeroe in het Tibetaans Tantrisme (The Guru in Tibetan Tantrism) – Erik Bruijn
Master Poe-Tai, the happy wanderer – Erik Bruijn
Published by Ankh-Hermes B.V., Deventer

With thanks to Erik Bruijn for making wood engravings available from his own collection, from the pantheon of the Changcha Hutuktu and from the Narthang pantheon.

Alphabetical Index

Also published in this series

Eva Rudy Jansen

The Book of Hindu Imagery
The Gods and their Symbols

Hinduism is more than a religion; it is a way of life that has developed over approximately 5 millennia. Its rich history has made the structure of its mythical and philosophical principles into a highly differentiated maze, of wich total knowledge is a practical impossibility. This volume cannot offer a complete survey of the meaning of Hinduism, but it does provide an extensive compilation of important deities and their divine manifestations, so that modern students van understand the Hindu pantheon. To facilitate easy recognition, a survey of ritual gestures, postures, attires and attributes, and an index are included

ISBN 90-74597-07-6

Ab Williams

The Complete Book of Chinese Health Balls
Practical Exercises

This book deals with an ancient Chinese fitness technique that has been in use since the Ming Dynasty (1368-1644). Two, usually metal, balls are to be moved around in the palm of the hand, thus stimulating the nervous system. These health balls are believed to improve memory, stimulate circulation, relax the muscles and tune the chi (life energy). In this book you will learn about chi and the nervous system and you will find a wide range of practical exercises that will enable you to optimise your energy. The author discusses the historical backgrounds, gives a survey of the different types of balls and their characteristics and takes you step-by-step through the basic exercises, walking and meditation exercises, and teaches you how to use the balls for massage and for strengthening and balacing the ying/yang energy in your body.

ISBN 90-74597-03-3

George Hulskramer

The Life of Buddha
From Prince Siddharta to Buddha

There are few histories of Prince Siddharta that are as accessible to all ages as this one. In comic-book format, Hulskramer tells the colorful story of the Buddha Siddharta, skillfully illustrated by Nepalese artists Raju Babu Shakya and Bijay Raj Shakya. This is a readable biography for anyone who is interested in Buddhism, a wonderful, exotic fairytale for lovers of beautiful illustrated stories, and a collector's item for cartoon enthusiasts.

ISBN 90-74597-17-3

Töm Klöwer

The Joy of Drumming
Drums en Percussion Instruments from around the World

This book is an appeal for a rediscovery of the spiritual and physical healing potential of rhythmic sound, and for the importance of musical creativity in our daily lives. Klöwer discusses how different cultures from around the world have used percussion in their spiritual practices for healing and conflict resolution, in communication, and for maintaining a sense of freedom and integrity. Everyone is creative and has musical potential, begin your fulfilling journey with this book.

The book includes over *100 illustrations of different drums, gongs, and sound effect instruments,* along with descriptions of how they are made, and basic playing techniques. From the most ancient instruments to the most modern inventions, from *Asia, Australia, Africa, and South America,* one of these instruments is sure to capture your imagination.

ISBN 90-74597-13-9

Dirk Schellberg

Didgeridoo
Ritual Origins and Playing Techniques

The didgeridoo plays an important role in the creation myths of the Australian Aborigines. The deep sound of this wind instrument helped create the world. This book describes the origins of the didgeridoo, the stories about the instrument and the players. It not only deals with Australian musicians and bands, but also discusses how Western therapists have discoverd new applications for this ancient sound. Also shows how to build an instrument, or what to look for in puchasing one.

ISBN 90-74597-13-0

Eva Rudy Jansen

Singing Bowls
A Practical Handbook of Instruction and Use

The Himalayan singing bowls, also known as Tibetan or Nepalese singing bowls, are a phenomenon which is facinating more and more westerners with the singing sound of the metal bowls. By going to concerts, undergoing so-called 'soundmassages' and by experimenting themselves, people discover all sorts of possibilities and aspects of these special sounds.

This book explores these possibilities and aspects, tells something about the backgrounds, and provides practical information about the ways in which the bowls can be played, and how to choose a bowl for oneself.

It also contains an extra chapter describing three other ritual objects: tingshaws (small cymbals), dorje (thunderbolt) and bell.

ISBN 90-74597-01-7